SOMATIC THERAPY FOR TRAUMA

Essential Manual To Unlock Natural Resilience With Mind-Body Techniques, And Nervous System Regulation

DR. MELISSA STOTLER

Copyright © 2023 by Dr. Melissa Stotler

Disclaimer:

The data in this book is solely meant to be informative and instructional.

This book is not intended to replace expert medical advice, diagnosis, or care. No medical, health, or other professional services are offered by the author, publisher, or any affiliated parties

Individual outcomes may differ in the practice of these therapies, which entail a variety of approaches and methodologies.

A one-on-one session with a trained or certified healthcare professional is still preferable. It is best to consult a trained healthcare provider before making any decisions regarding your health.

The author of this book is not affiliated with any specific website, product, or organization related to any of these therapies.

All reasonable measures have been taken by the author and publisher to guarantee the authenticity and dependability of the material contained in this book.

Contents

Somatic Therapy for Trauma offers a profound exploration into healing through the body, highlighting the critical intersection of physical and emotional well-being. This book provides an in-depth look at somatic therapy, tracing its historical roots and illustrating its evolution as a powerful tool for trauma recovery. Readers will gain a comprehensive understanding of various somatic approaches and the fundamental principles and techniques that underpin this therapeutic method. The benefits of somatic therapy in trauma healing are clearly articulated, emphasizing how this practice helps individuals reclaim their sense of safety and control.

Central to the healing process is the exploration of the body's response to trauma. The book delves into the fight, flight, and freeze responses, explaining how trauma manifests and is stored within the body. The nervous system's pivotal role in this process is detailed, along with the somatic symptoms that may arise. Readers are guided to recognize and address these symptoms, underscoring the importance of body awareness in the therapeutic journey.

Grounding techniques are highlighted as essential tools for managing trauma. The text elaborates on the concept of grounding, providing practical exercises that can be integrated into daily life to enhance stability and manage trauma triggers. These techniques are positioned as foundational in creating a sense of safety and continuity throughout the healing process.

The book also covers somatic experiences, offering a step-by-step guide to this technique.

It includes insights on how to release trauma stored in the body, utilizing methods such as titration and pendulation. Real-life case studies illustrate the effectiveness of somatic experiencing, enriching the reader's understanding of its application.

Breathwork is another vital component discussed, exploring its connection to trauma and various techniques for its application in somatic therapy. The benefits of conscious breathing are emphasized, with practical exercises provided to support trauma recovery.

Movement and its role in trauma release are thoroughly examined, presenting simple exercises to incorporate into daily routines. This section highlights how movement can facilitate reconnection with the body and promote healing, supported by success stories that showcase its transformative power.

Mindfulness and body awareness are woven throughout the narrative, with a focus on developing these practices to support trauma recovery. Readers are guided through mindful exercises and their role in regulating emotions, reinforcing the integration of mindfulness into everyday life.

Finally, the book addresses the integration of somatic therapy into daily living, offering strategies to continue healing outside of therapy. It provides guidance on establishing a daily somatic practice, building a support system, and overcoming challenges, celebrating the progress made along the way. This comprehensive guide is designed to empower individuals to sustain their healing journey and embrace continued growth and recovery.

Introduction To Somatic Therapy For Trauma

Somatic therapy is an innovative and holistic approach to trauma healing that emphasizes the connection between the mind and body. Unlike traditional talk therapies, which focus primarily on verbal expression and cognitive processes, somatic therapy integrates the physical experiences of the body into the healing process. This form of therapy acknowledges that trauma is not only a psychological event but also a physical one, where the body stores traumatic memories and responses. By addressing both the mind and body, somatic therapy offers a comprehensive pathway to recovery, helping individuals process and release trauma that may be trapped in their physical being.

Overview of Somatic Therapy

Somatic therapy is grounded in the understanding that our bodies hold onto experiences, especially those that are traumatic or stressful. This therapeutic approach works on the premise that trauma can cause disruptions in the body's natural functioning, leading to physical symptoms, chronic pain, and emotional distress. Somatic therapy aims to restore balance by facilitating awareness of bodily sensations and encouraging the release of stored tension. Through various techniques, individuals learn to reconnect with their bodies, recognize the impact of trauma on their physical state, and develop healthier ways to cope and heal.

One of the core elements of somatic therapy is the focus on body awareness. Clients are guided to notice and describe their physical sensations, such as tightness, tingling, or heaviness. This awareness allows them to connect these sensations to their emotional experiences, creating a bridge between the mind and body. By tuning into the body's signals, individuals can begin to understand how trauma has affected them on a physical level and start the process of releasing these effects.

Historical Background of Somatic Therapy

Somatic therapy has its roots in various body-centered healing practices that date back to ancient times, but it has evolved significantly over the last century. The modern development of somatic therapy can be traced to the work of Wilhelm Reich, an Austrian psychoanalyst who introduced the concept of "body armor" in the 1930s. Reich believed that the body stored repressed emotions and that releasing these emotions through physical movement could lead to psychological healing.

In the 1970s, Peter Levine, a pioneering therapist, expanded on Reich's ideas by developing Somatic Experiencing, a specific approach to trauma therapy. Levine observed that animals in the wild naturally discharged the energy generated by traumatic events, allowing them to recover without long-term effects. He theorized that humans could benefit from a similar process, which involves gradually releasing the energy associated with trauma stored in the body. Levine's work has been instrumental in shaping the field of somatic therapy as we know it today.

Over time, somatic therapy has continued to evolve, incorporating insights from various disciplines, including psychology, neuroscience, and Eastern healing traditions. This multidisciplinary approach has enriched somatic therapy, making it a versatile and effective method for addressing trauma.

Types of Somatic Approaches

Somatic therapy encompasses a range of approaches, each with its own unique techniques and theoretical foundations. These approaches share a common goal of integrating the body into the healing process, but they differ in their methods and focus areas.

Somatic Experiencing (SE):

Developed by Peter Levine, SE is one of the most well-known forms of somatic therapy. It focuses on helping individuals gradually release the energy and tension associated with trauma. Through a process called "pendulation," clients are guided to move between states of distress and calmness, allowing them to release traumatic energy in a controlled and safe manner.

Sensorimotor Psychotherapy:

This approach combines somatic therapy with traditional talk therapy, addressing both the physical and psychological aspects of trauma. Developed by Pat Ogden, Sensorimotor Psychotherapy emphasizes the importance of body awareness and movement in processing traumatic memories. It helps clients develop new, healthier physical responses to their emotions.

Bioenergetic Analysis:

Rooted in the work of Wilhelm Reich, Bioenergetic Analysis explores the relationship between the body and emotions. It involves physical exercises, such as grounding techniques and deep breathing, to help clients release stored emotions and increase their sense of vitality.

Hakomi Method:

The Hakomi Method, developed by Ron Kurtz, integrates mindfulness with body-centered therapy. This approach encourages clients to explore their inner experiences in a non-judgmental way, allowing them to uncover and address unconscious beliefs and patterns that may be contributing to their trauma.

Body-Mind Centering (BMC):

BMC is an approach that focuses on the exploration of movement and the body's systems, such as the nervous, muscular, and skeletal systems. Developed by Bonnie Bainbridge Cohen, BMC helps clients gain a deeper understanding of how their bodies hold and express trauma, facilitating healing through movement and awareness.

Key Principles and Techniques

Somatic therapy is based on several key principles that guide its practice. These principles emphasize the importance of body awareness, the integration of physical and emotional experiences, and the gradual release of traumatic energy.

Body Awareness:

One of the fundamental principles of somatic therapy is the focus on body awareness. Clients are encouraged to tune into their physical sensations and notice how their bodies respond to different emotions and experiences. This awareness helps individuals recognize the ways in which trauma has affected their bodies and begin the process of healing.

Grounding:

Grounding is a technique used in somatic therapy to help clients feel more connected to their bodies and the present moment. It involves practices such as deep breathing, mindfulness, and physical exercises that help individuals stay anchored in their bodies. Grounding techniques are particularly useful for clients who may feel disconnected or overwhelmed by their emotions.

Pendulation:

Pendulation is a technique developed by Peter Levine in Somatic Experiencing. It involves moving back and forth between states of distress and calmness, allowing clients to gradually release the energy associated with trauma. This process helps individuals build resilience and develop a greater capacity to tolerate difficult emotions.

Titration:

Titration is another technique used in somatic therapy, where clients are exposed to small, manageable doses of traumatic material. This gradual approach helps prevent clients from becoming overwhelmed and allows them to process and release trauma in a controlled and safe way.

Resourcing:

Resourcing involves identifying and cultivating internal and external resources that can provide comfort and support during the healing process. These resources might include positive memories, supportive relationships, or calming physical sensations. Resourcing helps clients build a sense of safety and stability as they work through their trauma.

Benefits of Somatic Therapy in Trauma Healing

Somatic therapy offers numerous benefits for individuals seeking to heal from trauma. By integrating the body into the therapeutic process, somatic therapy provides a holistic approach to healing that can lead to profound and lasting change.

Releasing Stored Trauma:

One of the primary benefits of somatic therapy is its ability to help individuals release trauma that has been stored in the body. Through techniques such as pendulation, titration, and body awareness, clients can gradually release the tension and energy associated with traumatic experiences. This release can lead to a reduction in physical symptoms, such as chronic pain, and an overall sense of relief and lightness.

Improved Emotional Regulation:

Somatic therapy helps clients develop greater awareness of their physical and emotional states, which can lead to improved emotional regulation. By learning to recognize and respond to their body's signals, individuals can develop healthier ways to cope with stress and difficult emotions. This increased emotional regulation can lead to greater resilience and a stronger sense of well-being.

Enhanced Mind-Body Connection:

Somatic therapy fosters a deeper connection between the mind and body, helping individuals develop a greater sense of self-awareness and self-compassion. This enhanced mind-body connection can lead to a more integrated and holistic sense of self, where individuals feel more in tune with their bodies and emotions.

Increased Sense of Safety:

Trauma can leave individuals feeling unsafe and disconnected from their bodies. Somatic therapy helps clients rebuild a sense of safety by grounding them in their bodies and teaching them techniques to manage their physical and emotional responses. This increased sense of safety can provide a solid foundation for healing and growth.

Holistic Healing:

Somatic therapy offers a holistic approach to trauma healing that addresses both the physical and psychological aspects of trauma. By integrating the body into the healing process, somatic therapy provides a more comprehensive and effective path to recovery.

This holistic approach can lead to deeper and more lasting healing, as it addresses the root causes of trauma and supports the body's natural ability to heal.

CHAPTER ONE

THE BODY'S RESPONSE TO TRAUMA

When trauma occurs, the body undergoes a series of complex physiological changes designed to protect us from harm.

These changes are rooted in survival mechanisms that have evolved over millions of years.

 When faced with a threatening situation, our body instinctively reacts to ensure our safety, triggering a cascade of responses that can be felt physically, emotionally, and mentally.

During a traumatic event, the body's stress response is activated. This response is primarily driven by the release of stress hormones like adrenaline and cortisol.

These hormones prepare the body for immediate action, increasing heart rate, tightening muscles, and heightening alertness. This state of heightened arousal is crucial for survival in the face of danger, but when trauma is unresolved, the body can remain in this heightened state long after the event has passed.

Chronic activation of the body's stress response can lead to a variety of physical symptoms, including tension, pain, fatigue, and digestive issues.

 It can also impact emotional well-being, contributing to feelings of anxiety, irritability, and depression.

Understanding how the body responds to trauma is the first step in recognizing the profound impact trauma can have on overall health and well-being.

Understanding The Fight, Flight, Freeze Response

The fight, flight, freeze response is a critical survival mechanism that is automatically activated when we perceive danger. It involves three potential reactions: fighting the threat, fleeing from it, or freezing in place. Each response serves a specific purpose in the context of survival, but when trauma is unresolved, these responses can become ingrained patterns that are triggered by situations that may not actually be dangerous.

Fight: When the body perceives a threat, the immediate reaction might be to confront it head-on. The fight response is characterized by a surge of energy and aggression, which prepares the body to physically defend itself. This response can manifest in feelings of anger or irritability, and physically, it might present as muscle tension or clenched fists.

Flight: If the body determines that confronting the threat is too dangerous, the next instinct is to flee. The flight response involves an overwhelming urge to escape from the situation. Physically, this can be felt as a quickening of the heart rate, shortness of breath, or a need to run. Emotionally, it might lead to feelings of anxiety or panic.

Freeze: In some cases, the body's response to danger is to freeze. This response can occur when neither fight nor flight seems possible or safe. Freezing is the body's way of shutting down in the face of overwhelming fear. It can manifest as a feeling of numbness, dissociation, or being "stuck" in place. Recognizing the freeze response is important because it can be easily misunderstood as inaction or apathy when, in reality, it is a deeply ingrained survival response.

Understanding these responses helps individuals recognize patterns in their behavior and bodily reactions, providing insight into how past traumas may be influencing their current experiences.

How Trauma Is Stored In The Body

Trauma is not just a mental or emotional experience; it also has a profound impact on the body. When we experience trauma, the memories and emotions associated with the event can become embedded in our physical body. This is because the body and mind are deeply interconnected, and what happens to one can affect the other.

Trauma can be stored in the body in various ways. One common manifestation is muscle tension and pain. During a traumatic event, the body tenses up as a protective mechanism. If the trauma is not fully processed, this tension can become chronic, leading to persistent pain or discomfort in specific areas of the body, such as the neck, shoulders, or lower back.

Another way trauma is stored in the body is through the autonomic nervous system, which controls involuntary bodily functions like heart rate and digestion. Trauma can dysregulate this system, leading to symptoms such as digestive issues, headaches, or chronic fatigue. These symptoms are the body's way of signaling that it is still holding onto the trauma.

Trauma can also be stored in the body as emotional energy. Emotions like fear, anger, or sadness may not be fully expressed during a traumatic event, and instead, they become trapped in the body. This trapped energy can create a sense of unease or agitation, and over time, it can contribute to the development of physical and mental health issues.

Understanding how trauma is stored in the body is crucial for healing because it highlights the need for a holistic approach that addresses both the mind and the body in the recovery process.

The Role Of The Nervous System

The nervous system plays a central role in how the body responds to and processes trauma. It is composed of the central nervous system (the brain and spinal cord) and the peripheral nervous system (the network of nerves that branch out from the spinal cord to the rest of the body).

The autonomic nervous system, a part of the peripheral nervous system, is particularly important in understanding trauma.

The autonomic nervous system has two main branches: the sympathetic nervous system, which activates the body's fight or flight response, and the parasympathetic nervous system, which promotes relaxation and healing. In a healthy, balanced state, these two systems work together to help the body respond to stress and then return to a state of calm.

However, when a person experiences trauma, the sympathetic nervous system can become overactive, keeping the body in a state of hyperarousal.

This can lead to symptoms such as anxiety, insomnia, and a constant feeling of being "on edge."

On the other hand, some individuals may experience a dominance of the parasympathetic nervous system, leading to symptoms of dissociation, numbness, or depression.

Healing from trauma involves helping the nervous system find balance again. This can be achieved through practices that calm the sympathetic nervous system, such as deep breathing, meditation, and mindfulness.

It can also involve engaging the parasympathetic nervous system through activities that promote relaxation and connection, such as gentle movement, creative expression, and spending time in nature.

Understanding the role of the nervous system in trauma helps individuals recognize the physiological basis of their symptoms and empowers them to take steps toward healing.

Recognizing Somatic Symptoms Of Trauma

Somatic symptoms are physical manifestations of trauma that can appear long after the traumatic event has occurred. These symptoms are often the body's way of communicating that it is still holding onto unresolved trauma. Recognizing these symptoms is a crucial step in the healing process because it allows individuals to address the root cause of their physical discomfort.

Some common somatic symptoms of trauma include chronic pain, headaches, digestive issues, and fatigue. These symptoms may not have an obvious medical explanation and can persist despite conventional treatment. For example, a person who has experienced trauma might suffer from chronic back pain that does not respond to physical therapy or medication. This pain may be a manifestation of unresolved emotional tension stored in the body.

Somatic symptoms can also include sensations such as tightness in the chest, difficulty breathing, or a racing heart. These symptoms often occur when the body is triggered by a reminder of the trauma, even if the individual is not consciously aware of the trigger. For instance, a person might feel a sudden surge of anxiety or panic when they are in a situation that subconsciously reminds them of a past trauma.

Recognizing these somatic symptoms allows individuals to connect their physical experiences with their emotional and psychological history. This awareness is the first step towards healing because it helps individuals understand that their symptoms are not just in their minds—they are real, physical experiences that deserve attention and care.

The Importance Of Body Awareness In Healing

Body awareness is a key component of healing from trauma because it involves tuning into the body's sensations, emotions, and signals. This awareness allows individuals to reconnect with their bodies in a safe and compassionate way, which is essential for processing and releasing trauma.

Practices that cultivate body awareness, such as mindfulness, yoga, and somatic experiencing, help individuals become more attuned to their physical and emotional states.

Through these practices, individuals can learn to recognize the early signs of stress or discomfort in their bodies, allowing them to address these issues before they escalate.

Body awareness also helps individuals develop a greater sense of safety and control in their bodies. Trauma can often lead to feelings of disconnection or dissociation from the body, making it difficult to trust bodily sensations or emotions. By cultivating body awareness, individuals can begin to rebuild this trust, leading to a deeper sense of self-compassion and resilience.

Furthermore, body awareness can facilitate the release of stored trauma. When individuals are able to fully experience and acknowledge their physical sensations, they can begin to process the emotions and memories associated with their trauma. This process can lead to profound healing as the body releases the tension and energy that has been held for so long.

Overall, body awareness is a powerful tool in the healing process, allowing individuals to reclaim their bodies and move towards a state of wholeness and well-being.

CHAPTER TWO

GROUNDING TECHNIQUES IN SOMATIC THERAPY

What Is Grounding And Why It's Important

Grounding is a technique used in somatic therapy to help individuals connect with the present moment, particularly when they are feeling overwhelmed by emotions or memories related to trauma.

Essentially, grounding helps anchor a person in the here and now, which can be especially beneficial when dealing with distressing thoughts or feelings that might feel out of control. By focusing on the present and their physical sensations, individuals can create a sense of stability and safety, which is crucial for effective trauma recovery.

Grounding is important because it counteracts the feeling of being disconnected or dissociated from one's body and surroundings. When someone is grounded, they are more aware of their current environment and their body's sensations, rather than being lost in past trauma or future anxieties. This connection helps in reducing symptoms of anxiety, panic, and dissociation, providing a more stable emotional and psychological state.

Simple Grounding Exercises For Daily Use

Body Scan: Begin by sitting or lying down in a comfortable position. Close your eyes and take a few deep breaths. Slowly shift your attention to different parts of your body, starting from your toes and moving up to your head. Notice any sensations, areas of tension, or relaxation. This exercise helps in reconnecting with your body and identifying physical sensations.

5-4-3-2-1 Technique: Engage your senses by identifying five things you can see, four things you can touch, three things you can hear, two things you can smell, and one thing you can taste. This exercise helps bring your attention to the present moment and your surroundings.

Grounding Objects: Carry a small, comforting object with you, such as a smooth stone or a piece of fabric. When feeling overwhelmed, hold the object in your hand and focus on its texture, weight, and temperature. This can serve as a tangible connection to the present.

Breathing Exercises: Practice deep, diaphragmatic breathing. Inhale slowly through your nose for a count of four, hold your breath for a count of four, and exhale slowly through your mouth for a count of six. This simple exercise helps calm the nervous system and anchor you in the present.

Mindful Walking: Take a walk and pay close attention to each step. Feel the ground beneath your feet, notice the movement of your legs, and observe the rhythm of your breathing. Mindful walking helps in connecting with your body and the present moment.

How To Stay Grounded During Therapy

Staying grounded during therapy involves using specific strategies to maintain a sense of stability and safety throughout the session. Here are some practical tips:

Use Grounding Objects: Bring a small item to therapy that you can hold or touch when you start to feel overwhelmed. This can help remind you of the present moment and provide comfort.

Practice Mindful Breathing: Before and during the therapy session, use deep breathing techniques to keep yourself centered. Focus on your breath to help manage anxiety or stress that may arise.

Set Intentions: At the beginning of each session, set an intention for what you want to achieve or focus on. This can help create a sense of purpose and direction, keeping you grounded throughout the session.

Engage in Sensory Techniques: If you begin to feel disconnected, use sensory techniques like touching the texture of your clothing or listening to soothing background sounds. These can help bring you back to the present moment.

Take Breaks: If you find yourself becoming overwhelmed, it's okay to take short breaks during the session. Use these moments to practice grounding techniques and reestablish your connection with the present.

Using Grounding To Manage Trauma Triggers

Trauma triggers can cause intense emotional or physical reactions that may feel uncontrollable. Grounding techniques can be effective in managing these triggers by helping you stay connected to the present moment. Here's how to use grounding in this context:

Identify Triggers: Begin by recognizing specific triggers that affect you. Understanding what causes these reactions allows you to prepare and use grounding techniques effectively when needed.

Implement Grounding Exercises: When a trigger is encountered, use grounding exercises such as the 5-4-3-2-1 technique or mindful breathing to bring yourself back to the present. These exercises can help shift your focus away from the trigger and reduce its intensity.

Create a Grounding Plan: Develop a personalized plan that includes your preferred grounding techniques and strategies. Having this plan ready can make it easier to implement when you face triggers.

Practice Regularly: Consistent practice of grounding exercises can make them more effective when dealing with triggers. Incorporate these exercises into your daily routine to build resilience.

Seek Support: If managing triggers becomes challenging, consider discussing them with your therapist. They can help you refine your grounding techniques and provide additional strategies tailored to your needs.

The Role Of Grounding In Building Safety

Grounding plays a crucial role in establishing a sense of safety, which is fundamental for effective trauma recovery. Here's how grounding contributes to building safety:

Enhancing Body Awareness: Grounding helps you become more aware of your physical sensations and body's responses. This increased awareness can lead to a better understanding of how your body responds to stress and trauma, allowing you to address these responses more effectively.

Creating a Stable Foundation: By consistently practicing grounding techniques, you build a reliable foundation of safety and stability. This stability provides a safe base from which to explore and process traumatic experiences.

Reducing Overwhelm: Grounding techniques help manage feelings of being overwhelmed by providing immediate, practical methods to regain control and calm. This reduction in overwhelm contributes to a greater sense of safety.

Strengthening Emotional Resilience: Regular grounding practices can enhance emotional resilience by helping you stay centered during challenging moments. This resilience supports your ability to cope with trauma-related emotions and situations.

Fostering Trust in the Therapeutic Process: A sense of safety established through grounding can enhance trust in the therapeutic process. When you feel grounded, you are more likely to engage openly with your therapist and work through trauma effectively.

CHAPTER THREE

SOMATIC EXPERIENCING TECHNIQUES

Somatic Experiencing (SE) is a therapeutic approach designed to help individuals process and release trauma stored in the body.

This technique focuses on the body's sensations and physiological responses to address trauma symptoms.

The key techniques include body awareness, tracking bodily sensations, and completing unfinished actions.

Body Awareness involves tuning into physical sensations, such as tightness, warmth, or discomfort, and observing how they shift over time. This awareness helps identify areas where trauma might be held.

Tracking Bodily Sensations is the practice of paying close attention to changes in physical sensations and emotional states. This helps in understanding how the body reacts to stress or trauma.

Completing Unfinished Actions means allowing the body to complete movements or actions that were interrupted by trauma. This might involve physical exercises or movements that help release pent-up energy.

By integrating these techniques, individuals can begin to unravel and heal from the effects of trauma stored in their bodies.

Somatic Experiencing

Somatic Experiencing is a body-focused therapeutic approach developed by Dr. Peter Levine.

It is based on the understanding that trauma can manifest as physical tension and discomfort. This method encourages individuals to become more attuned to their body's sensations and responses to help resolve trauma.

The process involves gently guiding individuals to focus on their bodily experiences, allowing them to process and release trauma without being overwhelmed.

SE aims to restore the body's natural balance and resilience by facilitating the release of stored tension and emotions.

In practice, Somatic Experiencing helps clients navigate their inner experiences in a safe and controlled manner, making it easier to address and heal trauma from a physical and emotional standpoint.

Step-By-Step Guide To Somatic Experiencing

Step 1: Grounding and Centering Begin by helping the client establish a sense of grounding. This involves feeling the connection to the ground through their feet and sensing the support of the ground. Centering involves bringing focus to the present moment, allowing the client to feel more stable and secure.

Step 2: Body Awareness Guide the client to bring attention to their bodily sensations. Encourage them to notice areas of tension, discomfort, or unusual sensations. This might involve simple prompts like "What do you feel in your chest right now?" or "Where do you notice tightness in your body?"

Step 3: Tracking Sensations Help the client track and observe the changes in their sensations over time. This involves noting shifts in intensity, location, or type of sensations. Encourage the client to describe these changes without judgment.

Step 4: Gentle Exploration Once the client is comfortable with tracking, gently explore the sensations. Ask them to identify any emotions or memories associated with these sensations. This exploration should be done at a pace that feels manageable for the client.

Step 5: Completing Unfinished ActionsIf appropriate, guide the client to engage in physical movements or actions that might help complete the cycle of stress or trauma. This could involve gentle stretching or mimicking actions related to the trauma experience.

Step 6: Integration Conclude the session by helping the client integrate their experiences. This might involve discussing any insights gained or practicing relaxation techniques to reinforce the progress made.

How To Release Trauma Held In The Body

Understanding Trauma Storage Trauma can be stored in the body as physical tension, discomfort, or restricted movement. Recognizing this helps in addressing and releasing these stored experiences.

Practicing Body Awareness Encourage regular practice of body awareness exercises. This includes paying attention to areas of tension, noticing changes in sensation, and exploring these sensations in a safe manner.

Engaging in Movement Incorporate gentle physical activities such as stretching, yoga, or rhythmic movement. These activities can help release pent-up energy and tension associated with trauma.

Using Breathwork Breathing exercises can aid in releasing trauma. Deep, mindful breathing helps in calming the nervous system and easing physical tension.

Seeking Professional Guidance Consider working with a trained Somatic Experiencing practitioner. They can provide tailored techniques and support for safely addressing and releasing trauma.

The Role Of Titration And Pendulation

Titration refers to the process of breaking down the traumatic experience into smaller, more manageable parts. Instead of overwhelming the individual with the full intensity of their trauma, titration allows them to process small fragments of the experience at a time. This approach helps prevent retraumatization and facilitates gradual healing.

Pendulation Pendulation involves moving between states of discomfort and comfort.

This technique encourages the client to oscillate between exploring distressing sensations and returning to a state of calm or neutrality.

By doing this, the individual learns to tolerate and integrate their traumatic experiences without becoming overwhelmed.

Applying Titration and PendulationIn practice, titration and pendulation can be applied by guiding the client to briefly focus on distressing sensations or memories, followed by periods of relaxation or positive experiences.

This approach helps balance the emotional experience and promotes healing by preventing excessive stress responses.

Case Studies: Somatic Experiencing in Action

Case Study 1: Trauma from a Car Accident A client who experienced a severe car accident reported persistent physical tension and anxiety.

Through Somatic Experiencing, the client focused on body awareness and tracked sensations related to the accident. By gradually exploring these sensations and engaging in gentle movement, the client was able to release stored tension and reduce anxiety.

Case Study 2: Childhood Abuse A client with a history of childhood abuse struggled with chronic pain and emotional distress. Using Somatic Experiencing techniques, the client worked on identifying areas of tension and engaging in breathwork.

The gradual exploration of these sensations, combined with pendulation, helped the client process and integrate traumatic memories, leading to a significant reduction in pain and emotional distress.

Case Study 3: Post-Traumatic Stress A client experiencing post-traumatic stress disorder (PTSD) utilized Somatic Experiencing to address symptoms such as hypervigilance and dissociation. The client engaged in titration and pendulation, focusing on manageable parts of their trauma and alternating between distress and relaxation. This approach helped the client gain greater control over their stress responses and improved their overall well-being.

These case studies illustrate the effectiveness of Somatic Experiencing in addressing and resolving trauma by focusing on bodily sensations and gradually processing traumatic experiences.

CHAPTER FOUR

BREATHWORK AND SOMATIC THERAPY

Breathwork is a powerful tool within somatic therapy, a therapeutic approach that focuses on the connection between the body and mind to address trauma. This technique involves intentional and controlled breathing patterns to help individuals access and release stored emotional and physical tension. By integrating breathwork into somatic therapy, practitioners can facilitate a deeper sense of relaxation and self-awareness, which is crucial for trauma recovery.

Breathwork techniques are used to regulate the autonomic nervous system, which plays a significant role in how we experience and respond to stress and trauma. Through various breathing exercises, individuals can activate the parasympathetic nervous system, promoting a state of calm and safety. This shift helps to counteract the hyperarousal often experienced by trauma survivors, allowing them to process and integrate their experiences more effectively.

The Connection Between Breath And Trauma

Trauma can significantly impact the way we breathe. Individuals who have experienced trauma often develop shallow or irregular breathing patterns as a result of chronic stress and hypervigilance.

This altered breathing pattern can contribute to physical symptoms such as tension, pain, and fatigue, as well as emotional difficulties like anxiety and depression.

Breathwork helps to reestablish a natural and balanced breathing rhythm, which is essential for restoring physical and emotional equilibrium.

By focusing on the breath, individuals can begin to break the cycle of stress and tension, creating a more conducive environment for healing.

Additionally, conscious breathing can help individuals become more aware of their body's responses to stress, facilitating a better understanding of how trauma manifests in their physical sensations.

Types Of Breathwork Techniques

There are several types of breathwork techniques used in somatic therapy, each with its unique approach and benefits. Some common techniques include:

Diaphragmatic Breathing: Also known as abdominal or deep breathing, this technique involves breathing deeply into the diaphragm rather than shallowly into the chest.

It helps to activate the parasympathetic nervous system, promoting relaxation and reducing stress.

Box Breathing: This technique involves inhaling, holding the breath, exhaling, and holding again, each for a count of four.

Box breathing helps to regulate the breath and calm the mind, making it a useful tool for managing anxiety and improving focus.

Holotropic Breathwork: Developed by Stanislav Grof, this technique involves rapid, deep breathing combined with evocative music and bodywork.

It aims to induce altered states of consciousness, allowing individuals to access and process deep-seated emotions and memories.

Alternate Nostril Breathing: This practice involves alternating the breath between the left and right nostrils.

 It is believed to balance the body's energy systems and promote mental clarity and emotional stability.

How To Use Breathwork In Somatic Therapy

In somatic therapy, breathwork can be integrated in various ways to enhance the therapeutic process. Here are some practical approaches:

Assessment: Begin by assessing the individual's current breathing patterns and their relationship to their trauma. This can be done through observation and discussion, helping to identify any breathing-related issues.

Guided Sessions:

Lead the individual through guided breathwork sessions, focusing on different techniques based on their needs.

For example, diaphragmatic breathing can be used to promote relaxation, while holotropic breathwork may be employed to explore deeper emotional issues.

Body Awareness: Encourage individuals to pay attention to how their breath affects their body. This can involve noticing areas of tension or discomfort that may be related to their trauma and using breathwork to release these sensations.

Integration: Help individuals integrate the insights and experiences gained from breathwork into their daily lives.

 This may involve incorporating breathwork practices into their self-care routines or using breathing techniques during stressful situations.

The Benefits Of Conscious Breathing For Trauma

Conscious breathing offers numerous benefits for individuals dealing with trauma. Some key advantages include:

Stress Reduction: By activating the parasympathetic nervous system, conscious breathing helps to reduce the body's stress response, leading to lower levels of anxiety and improved emotional well-being.

Enhanced Self-Awareness: Conscious breathing encourages individuals to tune into their bodily sensations and emotional states, fostering greater self-awareness and insight into how trauma affects them.

Improved Emotional Regulation: Regular practice of conscious breathing can help individuals manage their emotions more effectively, reducing the intensity of emotional reactions and promoting a sense of calm and stability.

Physical Relief: Breathing techniques can help alleviate physical symptoms associated with trauma, such as muscle tension, headaches, and fatigue, by promoting relaxation and reducing stress.

Practical Breathwork Exercises To Try

Here are some practical breathwork exercises that can be easily incorporated into daily life:

Deep Belly Breathing: Sit or lie down comfortably, placing one hand on your abdomen and the other on your chest.

Inhale deeply through your nose, allowing your abdomen to rise while keeping your chest still. Exhale slowly through your mouth, feeling your abdomen fall. Repeat for several minutes.

4-7-8 Breathing: Inhale quietly through your nose for a count of four, hold your breath for a count of seven, and exhale completely through your mouth for a count of eight. This exercise can be done several times a day to promote relaxation and reduce stress.

Progressive Muscle Relaxation with Breath: As you inhale deeply, tense a specific muscle group (such as your shoulders or hands).

Hold the tension for a few seconds, then exhale and release the tension. Move through different muscle groups, focusing on the sensation of relaxation with each breath.

Mindful Breathing: Take a few moments to sit quietly and focus solely on your breath. Observe the sensation of the breath entering and leaving your body without trying to change it. This exercise helps to cultivate mindfulness and a sense of calm.

By incorporating these techniques into your practice, you can effectively use breathwork to support trauma healing and promote overall well-being.

CHAPTER FIVE

MOVEMENT AND SOMATIC THERAPY

The Role Of Movement In Trauma Release

Movement plays a crucial role in somatic therapy by addressing trauma stored in the body. Trauma often manifests physically, resulting in tension, discomfort, or restricted movement.

Through intentional movement, individuals can begin to release these physical and emotional blockages.

The process works on the principle that the body holds onto traumatic experiences, and by moving deliberately, we can help shift these stored emotions.

This release allows for a deeper connection between mind and body, fostering healing and restoring balance.

Simple Movement Exercises For Trauma Healing

Engaging in simple movement exercises can be an effective way to facilitate trauma healing. One basic exercise is deep breathing combined with gentle stretching.

For instance, the "Cat-Cow Stretch" involves moving between arching and rounding the back while on hands and knees, which helps release tension along the spine.

Another useful exercise is the "Body Scan" where you lie down comfortably, focus on each part of your body, and consciously relax areas that feel tense.

These exercises, when practiced regularly, can help in releasing stored trauma and promoting a sense of calm and relaxation.

How To Integrate Movement Into Daily Life

Integrating movement into your daily routine can make it easier to address and manage trauma. Start by incorporating short movement breaks throughout the day.

For example, take a five-minute stretch break every hour if you're sitting for long periods. You can also use movement as a way to transition between tasks or when feeling stressed.

Simple activities like walking, stretching, or even dancing to your favorite music can help keep the body engaged and reduce tension. The key is to find movement practices that you enjoy and can maintain consistently, making them a natural part of your daily life.

Using Movement To Reconnect With The Body

Reconnecting with your body through movement involves becoming more aware of physical sensations and emotions. Practices such as mindful walking or body-centered yoga can enhance this connection.

During these activities, focus on how your body feels with each step or movement, and notice any areas of discomfort or ease. Techniques like "Body Awareness Meditation" can also help you tune into bodily sensations and emotions, fostering a deeper understanding of how trauma affects your physical state. This reconnection is essential for healing, as it helps you listen to and address the needs of your body.

Success Stories: Movement as a Healing Tool

Many individuals have found success in using movement as a tool for healing trauma. For example, people who have experienced trauma often report significant improvements in their emotional and physical well-being after incorporating somatic movement practices into their routines.

Stories abound of individuals who, through practices like yoga, dance, or tai chi, have managed to overcome chronic pain, anxiety, and depression related to their trauma.

These success stories highlight the transformative power of movement and its ability to support recovery, illustrating how engaging with one's body can lead to profound healing and personal growth.

CHAPTER SIX

MINDFULNESS AND BODY AWARENESS

What Is Mindfulness In Somatic Therapy?

Mindfulness in somatic therapy is the practice of maintaining a moment-to-moment awareness of our physical sensations, emotions, and thoughts.

It involves observing these experiences without judgment, allowing individuals to become more attuned to their internal states and responses.

This heightened awareness helps in recognizing patterns of stress and trauma stored in the body, leading to a more comprehensive understanding of one's experiences and needs.

In somatic therapy, mindfulness serves as a foundational tool to help clients connect with their bodily sensations, which can be crucial for healing trauma. By focusing on the present moment and observing bodily sensations as they arise, individuals can begin to notice how past traumas may be manifesting physically. This practice helps in identifying areas of tension or discomfort that may be related to unresolved issues, providing a pathway to address and heal these traumas.

Developing Body Awareness Through Mindfulness

Developing body awareness through mindfulness involves learning to tune into the physical sensations and signals your body is constantly sending.

This process requires training oneself to notice subtle changes in bodily sensations, such as muscle tension, changes in breathing patterns, or shifts in posture.

One effective way to enhance body awareness is through body scan meditations. In this practice, individuals lie down or sit comfortably and systematically focus their attention on different parts of the body.

Starting from the toes and moving upwards, the person observes any sensations without trying to change or judge them. This practice helps in recognizing areas of tension or discomfort and promotes a deeper connection with one's body.

Another method to build body awareness is through gentle movement practices, such as yoga or tai chi.

These activities encourage mindful movement and can help individuals become more aware of their physical presence and how their bodies respond to different movements and postures.

Mindful Practices To Support Trauma Recovery

Mindful practices can play a significant role in trauma recovery by fostering a safe and non-judgmental space for individuals to process their experiences.

One such practice is mindful breathing, which involves focusing on the breath as it enters and leaves the body. This practice helps calm the nervous system and can reduce symptoms of anxiety and stress.

Mindful walking is another technique where individuals practice walking slowly and attentively, paying close attention to each step and the sensations in their feet and legs.

This practice helps ground individuals in the present moment and can be particularly useful for those dealing with feelings of dissociation or being disconnected from their bodies.

Incorporating mindful journaling can also support trauma recovery. By writing down thoughts and feelings in a reflective and non-judgmental manner, individuals can gain insight into their emotional and physical experiences, facilitating a deeper understanding of their trauma and promoting healing.

The Role Of Mindfulness In Regulating Emotions

Mindfulness plays a crucial role in regulating emotions by enhancing one's ability to observe and understand emotional responses.

By practicing mindfulness, individuals can learn to identify their emotional triggers and recognize the early signs of emotional distress.

One of the key aspects of mindfulness is the ability to create space between stimulus and reaction. This space allows individuals to pause and choose how to respond to their emotions rather than reacting impulsively.

As a result, mindfulness helps in managing emotional responses more effectively and reduces the intensity of negative emotions.

Additionally, mindfulness can support emotional regulation by encouraging self-compassion.

By treating oneself with kindness and understanding during difficult emotional experiences, individuals can foster a more supportive internal environment, which contributes to emotional resilience and stability.

Exercises To Cultivate Mindfulness And Presence

Several exercises can help cultivate mindfulness and presence, making it easier to integrate these practices into daily life. One such exercise is mindful breathing, where individuals focus their attention on their breath, observing each inhale and exhale. This practice can be done for just a few minutes a day and helps center the mind and body.

Another effective exercise is mindful observation. In this practice, individuals choose an object, such as a candle or a flower, and observe it closely for a few minutes. They note the details, colors, textures, and any sensations or emotions that arise during the observation. This exercise helps enhance focus and brings attention to the present moment.

A simple yet powerful exercise is the "5-4-3-2-1" grounding technique. To practice this, individuals identify and name five things they can see, four things they can touch, three things they can hear, two things they can smell, and one thing they can taste.

This exercise helps anchor individuals in the present moment and can be particularly useful during times of stress or overwhelm.

CHAPTER SEVEN

INTEGRATING SOMATIC THERAPY INTO DAILY LIFE

Somatic therapy is not just a tool to be used during your sessions; it's a practice that can be woven into the fabric of your daily life.

By integrating somatic techniques into your routine, you can continue to heal, grow, and manage stress more effectively. One of the simplest ways to begin this integration is through mindful breathing.

Taking a few minutes each day to focus on your breath can help ground you in the present moment, reducing anxiety and bringing your awareness back to your body.

Another practical way to integrate somatic therapy is through body awareness exercises. These exercises involve paying close attention to the sensations in your body throughout the day. For example, while you're walking, notice how your feet feel against the ground, or when you're sitting, observe how your body feels supported by the chair.

This kind of mindful attention helps you stay connected to your body, which is crucial for healing trauma.

Additionally, incorporating movement into your daily life can enhance your somatic practice. This doesn't have to mean rigorous exercise; gentle stretching, yoga, or even dancing around your living room can be powerful ways to release stored tension and connect with your body.

The key is to move in ways that feel good and natural to you, allowing your body to guide you in what it needs.

How To Continue Healing Outside Of Therapy

Healing from trauma is an ongoing journey that doesn't end when you step out of your therapist's office. Continuing your healing process outside of therapy involves staying connected to the practices you've learned during your sessions. One effective strategy is to keep a journal where you can reflect on your experiences, track your progress, and note any triggers or emotions that arise. This practice helps you stay mindful of your healing journey and provides a safe space to process your thoughts and feelings.

Another important aspect of continuing your healing is practicing self-compassion. Trauma can often lead to harsh self-criticism, but learning to treat yourself with kindness and understanding is essential for recovery.

Whenever you notice negative self-talk, gently challenge it and replace it with affirmations that reinforce your worth and resilience.

In addition, maintaining a routine that supports your emotional and physical well-being is crucial. This might include regular exercise, healthy eating, adequate sleep, and engaging in activities that bring you joy and relaxation. By prioritizing your self-care, you create a strong foundation for ongoing healing.

Creating A Daily Somatic Practice

Establishing a daily somatic practice can significantly enhance your healing process by keeping you connected to your body and emotions. Start by setting aside a few minutes each day for a somatic exercise, such as body scanning. This involves mentally scanning your body from head to toe, paying attention to any areas of tension, discomfort, or numbness. As you become aware of these sensations, you can use your breath to release tension or simply acknowledge what your body is experiencing.

Another valuable daily practice is grounding. This technique helps anchor you in the present moment, especially when you're feeling overwhelmed or disconnected. Grounding can be as simple as standing barefoot on the earth, feeling the texture of the ground beneath your feet, or placing your hands on a solid surface and focusing on the sensation. These small but powerful actions can help you feel more stable and secure throughout your day.

It's also beneficial to incorporate movement into your daily somatic practice. Whether it's a few minutes of stretching in the morning, a walk during your lunch break, or a dance session at home, movement helps release stored energy and keeps you connected to your body. The key is consistency—by making these practices a regular part of your routine, they become second nature and support your ongoing healing.

Building A Support System For Ongoing Healing

Having a strong support system is crucial for anyone healing from trauma. This network can include friends, family, support groups, or even online communities where you feel safe and understood. The first step in building this system is to identify people in your life who are empathetic, trustworthy, and willing to support your healing journey. It's important to communicate your needs clearly to them, whether that's simply having someone to listen, or needing assistance with practical tasks when you're feeling overwhelmed.

Joining a support group, whether in person or online, can also be incredibly beneficial. These groups provide a space to share your experiences with others who understand what you're going through. Being part of such a community can help reduce feelings of isolation and give you a sense of belonging, which is vital for healing.

In addition to your personal network, consider seeking professional support when needed. This might involve continuing therapy, seeking out a somatic practitioner, or engaging in other therapeutic modalities that complement your healing process. Having multiple layers of support ensures that you have resources to draw on, no matter what challenges arise.

Overcoming Challenges In Somatic Healing

The journey of somatic healing is not always straightforward. You may encounter obstacles such as resistance, emotional overwhelm, or physical discomfort. Recognizing these challenges as a normal part of the healing process is important.

One common challenge is resistance to feeling difficult emotions. Trauma often leads to disconnection from the body as a protective mechanism, and reconnecting can sometimes bring up intense feelings.

When this happens, it's crucial to approach yourself with patience and compassion, allowing yourself to experience emotions at your own pace.

Another challenge is dealing with physical discomfort that may arise during somatic practices. This discomfort is often a sign that your body is releasing stored tension or trauma. Rather than avoiding these sensations, try to explore them with curiosity, noticing where they originate and how they change over time. Remember that it's okay to take breaks and that healing doesn't have to happen all at once.

It's also common to experience setbacks or periods where progress seems slow. During these times, it's important to stay committed to your practice and remind yourself that healing is a non-linear process.

Celebrate the small victories and understand that each step forward, no matter how small, is a significant part of your journey.

Celebrating Progress And Moving Forward

Celebrating your progress is an essential aspect of somatic healing. It's easy to focus on what still needs healing, but acknowledging how far you've come is equally important. Take time to reflect on the changes you've noticed in your body, emotions, and overall well-being. These might include reduced anxiety, better sleep, increased body awareness, or simply feeling more at peace. Recognizing these achievements helps reinforce your commitment to the healing process and boosts your confidence.

Another way to celebrate progress is by rewarding yourself for the work you've done. This could be as simple as treating yourself to a favorite activity, spending time with loved ones, or enjoying a day of relaxation. These rewards serve as reminders that your healing journey is worth celebrating and that you deserve to enjoy the fruits of your labor.

As you continue to move forward, it's important to set new goals for your healing journey. These goals don't have to be grand—they can be as simple as maintaining your daily somatic practice, continuing to build your support system, or exploring new therapeutic techniques. By setting these intentions, you keep your healing journey dynamic and forward-moving, always striving for greater well-being and self-awareness.

www.ingramcontent.com/pod-product-compliance
Lightning Source LLC
Chambersburg PA
CBHW061251250726
48653CB00002B/607